Strain

Grower _____ Date _____

Acquired _____ $ _____

Indica	Hybrid	Sativa

☐ Flower ☐ Edible ☐ Concentrate

Symptoms Relieved

_____
_____
_____
_____
_____

Sweet
Fruity   Floral
Sour   Spicy
Earthy   Herbal
Woodsy

Notes

_____
_____
_____
_____
_____
_____
_____

Effects	Strength				
Peaceful	○	○	○	○	○
Sleepy	○	○	○	○	○
Pain Relief	○	○	○	○	○
Hungry	○	○	○	○	○
Uplifted	○	○	○	○	○
Creative	○	○	○	○	○

Ratings ☆ ☆ ☆ ☆ ☆

Strain

Grower _____ Date _____

Acquired _____ $ _____

| Indica | Hybrid | Sativa |

☐ Flower ☐ Edible ☐ Concentrate

Symptoms Relieved

_____

_____

_____

_____

_____

Sweet

Fruity   Floral

Sour   Spicy

Earthy   Herbal

Woodsy

Notes

_____

_____

_____

_____

_____

_____

_____

Effects	Strength
Peaceful	○ ○ ○ ○ ○
Sleepy	○ ○ ○ ○ ○
Pain Relief	○ ○ ○ ○ ○
Hungry	○ ○ ○ ○ ○
Uplifted	○ ○ ○ ○ ○
Creative	○ ○ ○ ○ ○

Ratings ☆ ☆ ☆ ☆ ☆

Strain

Grower _____ Date _____

Acquired _____ $ _____

| Indica | Hybrid | Sativa |

☐ Flower ☐ Edible ☐ Concentrate

Symptoms Relieved

_____
_____
_____
_____
_____

Sweet
Fruity · Floral
Sour · Spicy
Earthy · Herbal
Woodsy

Notes

_____
_____
_____
_____
_____
_____

Effects	Strength
Peaceful	○ ○ ○ ○ ○
Sleepy	○ ○ ○ ○ ○
Pain Relief	○ ○ ○ ○ ○
Hungry	○ ○ ○ ○ ○
Uplifted	○ ○ ○ ○ ○
Creative	○ ○ ○ ○ ○

Ratings ☆ ☆ ☆ ☆ ☆

Strain

Grower _____   Date _____

Acquired _____ $ _____

| Indica | Hybrid | Sativa |

☐ Flower   ☐ Edible   ☐ Concentrate

Symptoms Relieved

_____

_____

_____

_____

_____

Sweet
Fruity   Floral
Sour   Spicy
Earthy   Herbal
Woodsy

Notes

_____

_____

_____

_____

_____

_____

_____

Effects	Strength				
Peaceful	○	○	○	○	○
Sleepy	○	○	○	○	○
Pain Relief	○	○	○	○	○
Hungry	○	○	○	○	○
Uplifted	○	○	○	○	○
Creative	○	○	○	○	○

Ratings ☆ ☆ ☆ ☆ ☆

Strain

Grower _____ Date _____

Acquired _____ $ _____

| Indica | Hybrid | Sativa |

☐ Flower   ☐ Edible   ☐ Concentrate

Symptoms Relieved

_____
_____
_____
_____
_____

Sweet
Fruity   Floral
Sour   Spicy
Earthy   Herbal
Woodsy

Notes

_____
_____
_____
_____
_____
_____
_____

Effects	Strength				
Peaceful	○	○	○	○	○
Sleepy	○	○	○	○	○
Pain Relief	○	○	○	○	○
Hungry	○	○	○	○	○
Uplifted	○	○	○	○	○
Creative	○	○	○	○	○

Ratings ☆ ☆ ☆ ☆ ☆

Strain

Grower _____ Date _____

Acquired _____ $ _____

| Indica | Hybrid | Sativa |

☐ Flower ☐ Edible ☐ Concentrate

Symptoms Relieved

_____
_____
_____
_____
_____

Sweet

Fruity   Floral

Sour   Spicy

Earthy   Herbal

Woodsy

Notes

_____
_____
_____
_____
_____
_____

Effects	Strength
Peaceful	○ ○ ○ ○ ○
Sleepy	○ ○ ○ ○ ○
Pain Relief	○ ○ ○ ○ ○
Hungry	○ ○ ○ ○ ○
Uplifted	○ ○ ○ ○ ○
Creative	○ ○ ○ ○ ○

Ratings ☆ ☆ ☆ ☆ ☆

Strain

Grower _____   Date _____

Acquired _____ $ _____

Indica	Hybrid	Sativa

☐ Flower   ☐ Edible   ☐ Concentrate

Symptoms Relieved

_____

_____

_____

_____

_____

Sweet

Fruity — Floral

Sour — Spicy

Earthy — Herbal

Woodsy

Notes

_____

_____

_____

_____

_____

_____

_____

Effects	Strength				
Peaceful	○	○	○	○	○
Sleepy	○	○	○	○	○
Pain Relief	○	○	○	○	○
Hungry	○	○	○	○	○
Uplifted	○	○	○	○	○
Creative	○	○	○	○	○

Ratings ☆ ☆ ☆ ☆ ☆

Strain

Grower _____   Date _____

Acquired _____ $ _____

Indica	Hybrid	Sativa

☐ Flower ☐ Edible ☐ Concentrate

Symptoms Relieved

_____

_____

_____

_____

_____

Sweet

Fruity   Floral

Sour   Spicy

Earthy   Herbal

Woodsy

Notes

_____

_____

_____

_____

_____

_____

Effects	**Strength**				
Peaceful	○	○	○	○	○
Sleepy	○	○	○	○	○
Pain Relief	○	○	○	○	○
Hungry	○	○	○	○	○
Uplifted	○	○	○	○	○
Creative	○	○	○	○	○

Ratings ☆ ☆ ☆ ☆ ☆

Strain

Grower _____ Date _____

Acquired _____ $ _____

| Indica | Hybrid | Sativa |

☐ Flower ☐ Edible ☐ Concentrate

Symptoms Relieved

_____

_____

_____

_____

_____

Sweet

Fruity   Floral

Sour   Spicy

Earthy   Herbal

Woodsy

Notes

_____

_____

_____

_____

_____

_____

Effects	**Strength**				
Peaceful	○	○	○	○	○
Sleepy	○	○	○	○	○
Pain Relief	○	○	○	○	○
Hungry	○	○	○	○	○
Uplifted	○	○	○	○	○
Creative	○	○	○	○	○

Ratings ☆ ☆ ☆ ☆ ☆

Strain

Grower _____   Date _____

Acquired _____ $ _____

Indica	Hybrid	Sativa

☐ Flower   ☐ Edible   ☐ Concentrate

Symptoms Relieved

_____

_____

_____

_____

_____

Sweet

Fruity   Floral

Sour   Spicy

Earthy   Herbal

Woodsy

Notes

_____

_____

_____

_____

_____

_____

Effects	Strength				
Peaceful	○	○	○	○	○
Sleepy	○	○	○	○	○
Pain Relief	○	○	○	○	○
Hungry	○	○	○	○	○
Uplifted	○	○	○	○	○
Creative	○	○	○	○	○

Ratings ☆ ☆ ☆ ☆ ☆

Strain

Grower _____   Date _____

Acquired _____ $ _____

| Indica | Hybrid | Sativa |

☐ Flower   ☐ Edible   ☐ Concentrate

Symptoms Relieved

_____

_____

_____

_____

_____

Sweet
Fruity   Floral
Sour   Spicy
Earthy   Herbal
Woodsy

Notes

_____

_____

_____

_____

_____

_____

Effects	**Strength**				
Peaceful	○	○	○	○	○
Sleepy	○	○	○	○	○
Pain Relief	○	○	○	○	○
Hungry	○	○	○	○	○
Uplifted	○	○	○	○	○
Creative	○	○	○	○	○

Ratings ☆ ☆ ☆ ☆ ☆

Strain

Grower _____   Date _____

Acquired _____ $ _____

| Indica | Hybrid | Sativa |

☐ Flower   ☐ Edible   ☐ Concentrate

Symptoms Relieved

_____

_____

_____

_____

_____

Sweet

Fruity   Floral

Sour   Spicy

Earthy   Herbal

Woodsy

Notes

_____

_____

_____

_____

_____

_____

Effects	Strength				
Peaceful	○	○	○	○	○
Sleepy	○	○	○	○	○
Pain Relief	○	○	○	○	○
Hungry	○	○	○	○	○
Uplifted	○	○	○	○	○
Creative	○	○	○	○	○

Ratings ☆ ☆ ☆ ☆ ☆

Strain

Grower _____   Date _____

Acquired _____ $ _____

Indica	Hybrid	Sativa

☐ Flower   ☐ Edible   ☐ Concentrate

Symptoms Relieved

_____

_____

_____

_____

_____

Sweet
Fruity   Floral
Sour   Spicy
Earthy   Herbal
Woodsy

Notes

_____

_____

_____

_____

_____

_____

Effects	Strength				
Peaceful	○	○	○	○	○
Sleepy	○	○	○	○	○
Pain Relief	○	○	○	○	○
Hungry	○	○	○	○	○
Uplifted	○	○	○	○	○
Creative	○	○	○	○	○

Ratings ☆ ☆ ☆ ☆ ☆

Strain

Grower _____ Date _____

Acquired _____ $ _____

| Indica | Hybrid | Sativa |

☐ Flower ☐ Edible ☐ Concentrate

Symptoms Relieved

_____

_____

_____

_____

_____

Sweet

Fruity   Floral

Sour   Spicy

Earthy   Herbal

Woodsy

Notes

_____

_____

_____

_____

_____

_____

_____

Effects	Strength
Peaceful	○ ○ ○ ○ ○
Sleepy	○ ○ ○ ○ ○
Pain Relief	○ ○ ○ ○ ○
Hungry	○ ○ ○ ○ ○
Uplifted	○ ○ ○ ○ ○
Creative	○ ○ ○ ○ ○

Ratings ☆ ☆ ☆ ☆ ☆

Strain

Grower _____ Date _____

Acquired _____ $ _____

| Indica | Hybrid | Sativa |

☐ Flower ☐ Edible ☐ Concentrate

Symptoms Relieved

_____
_____
_____
_____
_____

Sweet

Fruity   Floral

Sour   Spicy

Earthy   Herbal

Woodsy

Notes

_____
_____
_____
_____
_____
_____

Effects	**Strength**				
Peaceful	○	○	○	○	○
Sleepy	○	○	○	○	○
Pain Relief	○	○	○	○	○
Hungry	○	○	○	○	○
Uplifted	○	○	○	○	○
Creative	○	○	○	○	○

Ratings ☆ ☆ ☆ ☆ ☆

Strain

Grower _____ Date _____

Acquired _____ $ _____

Indica	Hybrid	Sativa

☐ Flower   ☐ Edible   ☐ Concentrate

Symptoms Relieved

_____

_____

_____

_____

_____

Sweet
Fruity   Floral
Sour   Spicy
Earthy   Herbal
Woodsy

Notes

_____

_____

_____

_____

_____

_____

_____

Effects	Strength				
Peaceful	○	○	○	○	○
Sleepy	○	○	○	○	○
Pain Relief	○	○	○	○	○
Hungry	○	○	○	○	○
Uplifted	○	○	○	○	○
Creative	○	○	○	○	○

Ratings ☆ ☆ ☆ ☆ ☆

Strain

Grower _____   Date _____

Acquired _____ $ _____

Indica	Hybrid	Sativa

☐ Flower ☐ Edible ☐ Concentrate

Symptoms Relieved

_____

_____

_____

_____

_____

Sweet

Fruity   Floral

Sour   Spicy

Earthy   Herbal

Woodsy

Notes

_____

_____

_____

_____

_____

_____

_____

Effects	**Strength**				
Peaceful	○	○	○	○	○
Sleepy	○	○	○	○	○
Pain Relief	○	○	○	○	○
Hungry	○	○	○	○	○
Uplifted	○	○	○	○	○
Creative	○	○	○	○	○

Ratings ☆ ☆ ☆ ☆ ☆

Strain

Grower _____   Date _____

Acquired _____ $ _____

Indica	Hybrid	Sativa

☐ Flower   ☐ Edible   ☐ Concentrate

Symptoms Relieved

_____

_____

_____

_____

_____

Sweet
Fruity   Floral
Sour   Spicy
Earthy   Herbal
Woodsy

Notes

_____

_____

_____

_____

_____

_____

Effects		**Strength**			
Peaceful	○	○	○	○	○
Sleepy	○	○	○	○	○
Pain Relief	○	○	○	○	○
Hungry	○	○	○	○	○
Uplifted	○	○	○	○	○
Creative	○	○	○	○	○

Ratings ☆ ☆ ☆ ☆ ☆

Strain

Grower _____   Date _____

Acquired _____ $ _____

| Indica | Hybrid | Sativa |

☐ Flower   ☐ Edible   ☐ Concentrate

Symptoms Relieved

_____

_____

_____

_____

_____

Sweet

Fruity · Floral

Sour · Spicy

Earthy · Herbal

Woodsy

Notes

_____

_____

_____

_____

_____

_____

Effects	Strength				
Peaceful	○	○	○	○	○
Sleepy	○	○	○	○	○
Pain Relief	○	○	○	○	○
Hungry	○	○	○	○	○
Uplifted	○	○	○	○	○
Creative	○	○	○	○	○

Ratings ☆ ☆ ☆ ☆ ☆

Strain

Grower _____   Date _____

Acquired _____ $ _____

| Indica | Hybrid | Sativa |

☐ Flower   ☐ Edible   ☐ Concentrate

Symptoms Relieved

_____

_____

_____

_____

_____

Sweet

Fruity   Floral

Sour   Spicy

Earthy   Herbal

Woodsy

Notes

_____

_____

_____

_____

_____

_____

Effects	Strength				
Peaceful	○	○	○	○	○
Sleepy	○	○	○	○	○
Pain Relief	○	○	○	○	○
Hungry	○	○	○	○	○
Uplifted	○	○	○	○	○
Creative	○	○	○	○	○

Ratings ☆ ☆ ☆ ☆ ☆

Strain

Grower _____   Date _____

Acquired _____ $ _____

| Indica | Hybrid | Sativa |

☐ Flower   ☐ Edible   ☐ Concentrate

Symptoms Relieved

_____

_____

_____

_____

_____

Sweet
Fruity   Floral
Sour   Spicy
Earthy   Herbal
Woodsy

Notes

_____

_____

_____

_____

_____

_____

Effects	Strength				
Peaceful	○	○	○	○	○
Sleepy	○	○	○	○	○
Pain Relief	○	○	○	○	○
Hungry	○	○	○	○	○
Uplifted	○	○	○	○	○
Creative	○	○	○	○	○

Ratings ☆ ☆ ☆ ☆ ☆

Strain

Grower _____   Date _____

Acquired _____ $ _____

Indica	Hybrid	Sativa

☐ Flower   ☐ Edible   ☐ Concentrate

Symptoms Relieved

_____

_____

_____

_____

_____

Sweet
Fruity   Floral
Sour   Spicy
Earthy   Herbal
Woodsy

Notes

_____

_____

_____

_____

_____

_____

Effects	Strength				
Peaceful	○	○	○	○	○
Sleepy	○	○	○	○	○
Pain Relief	○	○	○	○	○
Hungry	○	○	○	○	○
Uplifted	○	○	○	○	○
Creative	○	○	○	○	○

Ratings ☆ ☆ ☆ ☆ ☆

Strain

_____

Grower _____ Date _____

Acquired _____ $ _____

| Indica | Hybrid | Sativa |

☐ Flower   ☐ Edible   ☐ Concentrate

Symptoms Relieved

_____

_____

_____

_____

_____

Sweet

Fruity   Floral

Sour   Spicy

Earthy   Herbal

Woodsy

Notes

_____

_____

_____

_____

_____

_____

Effects	Strength				
Peaceful	○	○	○	○	○
Sleepy	○	○	○	○	○
Pain Relief	○	○	○	○	○
Hungry	○	○	○	○	○
Uplifted	○	○	○	○	○
Creative	○	○	○	○	○

Ratings ☆ ☆ ☆ ☆ ☆

Strain

Grower _____   Date _____

Acquired _____ $ _____

| Indica | Hybrid | Sativa |

☐ Flower   ☐ Edible   ☐ Concentrate

Symptoms Relieved

_____

_____

_____

_____

_____

Sweet
Fruity
Floral
Sour
Spicy
Earthy
Herbal
Woodsy

Notes

_____

_____

_____

_____

_____

_____

Effects	Strength
Peaceful	◯ ◯ ◯ ◯ ◯
Sleepy	◯ ◯ ◯ ◯ ◯
Pain Relief	◯ ◯ ◯ ◯ ◯
Hungry	◯ ◯ ◯ ◯ ◯
Uplifted	◯ ◯ ◯ ◯ ◯
Creative	◯ ◯ ◯ ◯ ◯

Ratings ☆ ☆ ☆ ☆ ☆

Strain

Grower _____   Date _____

Acquired _____ $ _____

| Indica | Hybrid | Sativa |

☐ Flower   ☐ Edible   ☐ Concentrate

Symptoms Relieved

_____

_____

_____

_____

_____

Sweet

Fruity   Floral

Sour   Spicy

Earthy   Herbal

Woodsy

Notes

_____

_____

_____

_____

_____

_____

_____

Effects	Strength				
Peaceful	○	○	○	○	○
Sleepy	○	○	○	○	○
Pain Relief	○	○	○	○	○
Hungry	○	○	○	○	○
Uplifted	○	○	○	○	○
Creative	○	○	○	○	○

Ratings ☆ ☆ ☆ ☆ ☆

Strain

Grower _____ Date _____

Acquired _____ $ _____

Indica	Hybrid	Sativa

☐ Flower   ☐ Edible   ☐ Concentrate

Symptoms Relieved

_____

_____

_____

_____

_____

Sweet
Fruity   Floral
Sour   Spicy
Earthy   Herbal
Woodsy

Notes

_____

_____

_____

_____

_____

_____

Effects	Strength				
Peaceful	○	○	○	○	○
Sleepy	○	○	○	○	○
Pain Relief	○	○	○	○	○
Hungry	○	○	○	○	○
Uplifted	○	○	○	○	○
Creative	○	○	○	○	○

Ratings ☆ ☆ ☆ ☆ ☆

Strain

Grower _____   Date _____

Acquired _____ $ _____

| Indica | Hybrid | Sativa |

☐ Flower   ☐ Edible   ☐ Concentrate

Symptoms Relieved

_____

_____

_____

_____

_____

Sweet
Fruity   Floral
Sour   Spicy
Earthy   Herbal
Woodsy

Notes

_____

_____

_____

_____

_____

_____

_____

Effects	Strength				
Peaceful	○	○	○	○	○
Sleepy	○	○	○	○	○
Pain Relief	○	○	○	○	○
Hungry	○	○	○	○	○
Uplifted	○	○	○	○	○
Creative	○	○	○	○	○

Ratings ☆ ☆ ☆ ☆ ☆

Strain

Grower _____   Date _____

Acquired _____ $ _____

| Indica | Hybrid | Sativa |

☐ Flower ☐ Edible ☐ Concentrate

Symptoms Relieved

_____

_____

_____

_____

_____

Sweet
Fruity   Floral
Sour   Spicy
Earthy   Herbal
Woodsy

Notes

_____

_____

_____

_____

_____

_____

Effects	Strength				
Peaceful	◯	◯	◯	◯	◯
Sleepy	◯	◯	◯	◯	◯
Pain Relief	◯	◯	◯	◯	◯
Hungry	◯	◯	◯	◯	◯
Uplifted	◯	◯	◯	◯	◯
Creative	◯	◯	◯	◯	◯

Ratings ☆ ☆ ☆ ☆ ☆

Strain

Grower _____   Date _____

Acquired _____ $ _____

Indica	Hybrid	Sativa

☐ Flower   ☐ Edible   ☐ Concentrate

Symptoms Relieved

_____

_____

_____

_____

_____

Sweet

Fruity   Floral

Sour   Spicy

Earthy   Herbal

Woodsy

Notes

_____

_____

_____

_____

_____

_____

_____

Effects	**Strength**				
Peaceful	○	○	○	○	○
Sleepy	○	○	○	○	○
Pain Relief	○	○	○	○	○
Hungry	○	○	○	○	○
Uplifted	○	○	○	○	○
Creative	○	○	○	○	○

Ratings ☆ ☆ ☆ ☆ ☆

Strain

Grower _____   Date _____

Acquired _____ $ _____

Indica	Hybrid	Sativa

☐ Flower   ☐ Edible   ☐ Concentrate

Symptoms Relieved

_____

_____

_____

_____

_____

Sweet · Fruity · Floral · Spicy · Herbal · Woodsy · Earthy · Sour

Notes

_____

_____

_____

_____

_____

_____

Effects	Strength				
Peaceful	○	○	○	○	○
Sleepy	○	○	○	○	○
Pain Relief	○	○	○	○	○
Hungry	○	○	○	○	○
Uplifted	○	○	○	○	○
Creative	○	○	○	○	○

Ratings ☆ ☆ ☆ ☆ ☆

Strain

Grower _____   Date _____

Acquired _____ $ _____

| Indica | Hybrid | Sativa |

☐ Flower   ☐ Edible   ☐ Concentrate

Symptoms Relieved

_____

_____

_____

_____

_____

Sweet
Fruity   Floral
Sour   Spicy
Earthy   Herbal
Woodsy

Notes

_____

_____

_____

_____

_____

_____

Effects	Strength				
Peaceful	○	○	○	○	○
Sleepy	○	○	○	○	○
Pain Relief	○	○	○	○	○
Hungry	○	○	○	○	○
Uplifted	○	○	○	○	○
Creative	○	○	○	○	○

Ratings ☆ ☆ ☆ ☆ ☆

Strain

Grower _____   Date _____

Acquired _____ $ _____

| Indica | Hybrid | Sativa |

☐ Flower   ☐ Edible   ☐ Concentrate

Symptoms Relieved

_____

_____

_____

_____

_____

Sweet

Fruity   Floral

Sour   Spicy

Earthy   Herbal

Woodsy

Notes

_____

_____

_____

_____

_____

_____

_____

Effects	Strength				
Peaceful	○	○	○	○	○
Sleepy	○	○	○	○	○
Pain Relief	○	○	○	○	○
Hungry	○	○	○	○	○
Uplifted	○	○	○	○	○
Creative	○	○	○	○	○

Ratings ☆ ☆ ☆ ☆ ☆

Strain

Grower _____ Date _____

Acquired _____ $ _____

| Indica | Hybrid | Sativa |

☐ Flower ☐ Edible ☐ Concentrate

Symptoms Relieved

_____

_____

_____

_____

Sweet
Fruity   Floral
Sour   Spicy
Earthy   Herbal
Woodsy

Notes

_____

_____

_____

_____

_____

_____

Effects	Strength				
Peaceful	○	○	○	○	○
Sleepy	○	○	○	○	○
Pain Relief	○	○	○	○	○
Hungry	○	○	○	○	○
Uplifted	○	○	○	○	○
Creative	○	○	○	○	○

Ratings ☆ ☆ ☆ ☆ ☆

Strain

Grower _____   Date _____

Acquired _____ $ _____

| Indica | Hybrid | Sativa |

☐ Flower   ☐ Edible   ☐ Concentrate

Symptoms Relieved

_____

_____

_____

_____

_____

Sweet

Fruity   Floral

Sour   Spicy

Earthy   Herbal

Woodsy

Notes

_____

_____

_____

_____

_____

_____

Effects	**Strength**				
Peaceful	○	○	○	○	○
Sleepy	○	○	○	○	○
Pain Relief	○	○	○	○	○
Hungry	○	○	○	○	○
Uplifted	○	○	○	○	○
Creative	○	○	○	○	○

Ratings ☆ ☆ ☆ ☆ ☆

Strain

Grower _____ Date _____

Acquired _____ $ _____

| Indica | Hybrid | Sativa |

☐ Flower ☐ Edible ☐ Concentrate

Symptoms Relieved

_____
_____
_____
_____
_____

Sweet
Fruity
Floral
Sour
Spicy
Earthy
Herbal
Woodsy

Notes

_____
_____
_____
_____
_____
_____
_____

Effects	**Strength**				
Peaceful	○	○	○	○	○
Sleepy	○	○	○	○	○
Pain Relief	○	○	○	○	○
Hungry	○	○	○	○	○
Uplifted	○	○	○	○	○
Creative	○	○	○	○	○

Ratings ☆ ☆ ☆ ☆ ☆

Strain

Grower _____   Date _____

Acquired _____ $ _____

Indica	Hybrid	Sativa

☐ Flower ☐ Edible ☐ Concentrate

Symptoms Relieved

_____

_____

_____

_____

_____

Sweet
Fruity
Floral
Sour
Spicy
Earthy
Herbal
Woodsy

Notes

_____

_____

_____

_____

_____

_____

Effects	Strength				
Peaceful	◯	◯	◯	◯	◯
Sleepy	◯	◯	◯	◯	◯
Pain Relief	◯	◯	◯	◯	◯
Hungry	◯	◯	◯	◯	◯
Uplifted	◯	◯	◯	◯	◯
Creative	◯	◯	◯	◯	◯

Ratings ☆ ☆ ☆ ☆ ☆

Strain

Grower _____ Date _____

Acquired _____ $ _____

| Indica | Hybrid | Sativa |

☐ Flower ☐ Edible ☐ Concentrate

Symptoms Relieved

_____

_____

_____

_____

_____

Sweet

Fruity Floral

Sour Spicy

Earthy Herbal

Woodsy

Notes

_____

_____

_____

_____

_____

_____

_____

Effects	Strength				
Peaceful	○	○	○	○	○
Sleepy	○	○	○	○	○
Pain Relief	○	○	○	○	○
Hungry	○	○	○	○	○
Uplifted	○	○	○	○	○
Creative	○	○	○	○	○

Ratings ☆ ☆ ☆ ☆ ☆

Strain

Grower _____   Date _____

Acquired _____ $ _____

| Indica | Hybrid | Sativa |

☐ Flower ☐ Edible ☐ Concentrate

Symptoms Relieved

_____

_____

_____

_____

_____

Sweet
Fruity   Floral
Sour   Spicy
Earthy   Herbal
Woodsy

Notes

_____

_____

_____

_____

_____

_____

_____

Effects	Strength				
Peaceful	○	○	○	○	○
Sleepy	○	○	○	○	○
Pain Relief	○	○	○	○	○
Hungry	○	○	○	○	○
Uplifted	○	○	○	○	○
Creative	○	○	○	○	○

Ratings ☆ ☆ ☆ ☆ ☆

Strain

Grower _____ Date _____

Acquired _____ $ _____

| Indica | Hybrid | Sativa |

☐ Flower   ☐ Edible   ☐ Concentrate

Symptoms Relieved

_____

_____

_____

_____

_____

Sweet
Fruity   Floral
Sour   Spicy
Earthy   Herbal
Woodsy

Notes

_____

_____

_____

_____

_____

_____

Effects	Strength				
Peaceful	○	○	○	○	○
Sleepy	○	○	○	○	○
Pain Relief	○	○	○	○	○
Hungry	○	○	○	○	○
Uplifted	○	○	○	○	○
Creative	○	○	○	○	○

Ratings ☆ ☆ ☆ ☆ ☆

Strain

Grower _____ Date _____

Acquired _____ $ _____

| Indica | Hybrid | Sativa |

☐ Flower ☐ Edible ☐ Concentrate

Symptoms Relieved

_____

_____

_____

_____

_____

Sweet
Fruity   Floral
Sour   Spicy
Earthy   Herbal
Woodsy

Notes

_____

_____

_____

_____

_____

_____

Effects	Strength				
Peaceful	○	○	○	○	○
Sleepy	○	○	○	○	○
Pain Relief	○	○	○	○	○
Hungry	○	○	○	○	○
Uplifted	○	○	○	○	○
Creative	○	○	○	○	○

Ratings ☆ ☆ ☆ ☆ ☆

Strain

Grower _____ Date _____

Acquired _____ $ _____

| Indica | Hybrid | Sativa |

☐ Flower   ☐ Edible   ☐ Concentrate

Symptoms Relieved

_____

_____

_____

_____

_____

Sweet

Fruity   Floral

Sour   Spicy

Earthy   Herbal

Woodsy

Notes

_____

_____

_____

_____

_____

_____

_____

Effects	**Strength**				
Peaceful	○	○	○	○	○
Sleepy	○	○	○	○	○
Pain Relief	○	○	○	○	○
Hungry	○	○	○	○	○
Uplifted	○	○	○	○	○
Creative	○	○	○	○	○

Ratings ☆ ☆ ☆ ☆ ☆

Strain

Grower _____ Date _____

Acquired _____ $ _____

| Indica | Hybrid | Sativa |

☐ Flower ☐ Edible ☐ Concentrate

Symptoms Relieved

_____

_____

_____

_____

_____

Sweet

Fruity

Floral

Sour

Spicy

Earthy

Herbal

Woodsy

Notes

_____

_____

_____

_____

_____

_____

Effects	Strength
Peaceful	○ ○ ○ ○ ○
Sleepy	○ ○ ○ ○ ○
Pain Relief	○ ○ ○ ○ ○
Hungry	○ ○ ○ ○ ○
Uplifted	○ ○ ○ ○ ○
Creative	○ ○ ○ ○ ○

Ratings ☆ ☆ ☆ ☆ ☆

Strain

Grower _____ Date _____

Acquired _____ $ _____

Indica	Hybrid	Sativa

☐ Flower ☐ Edible ☐ Concentrate

Symptoms Relieved

_____

_____

_____

_____

_____

Sweet

Fruity   Floral

Sour   Spicy

Earthy   Herbal

Woodsy

Notes

_____

_____

_____

_____

_____

_____

Effects	Strength				
Peaceful	○	○	○	○	○
Sleepy	○	○	○	○	○
Pain Relief	○	○	○	○	○
Hungry	○	○	○	○	○
Uplifted	○	○	○	○	○
Creative	○	○	○	○	○

Ratings ☆ ☆ ☆ ☆ ☆

Strain

Grower _____ Date _____

Acquired _____ $ _____

| Indica | Hybrid | Sativa |

☐ Flower ☐ Edible ☐ Concentrate

Symptoms Relieved

_____

_____

_____

_____

_____

Sweet

Fruity   Floral

Sour   Spicy

Earthy   Herbal

Woodsy

Notes

_____

_____

_____

_____

_____

_____

Effects	Strength				
Peaceful	○	○	○	○	○
Sleepy	○	○	○	○	○
Pain Relief	○	○	○	○	○
Hungry	○	○	○	○	○
Uplifted	○	○	○	○	○
Creative	○	○	○	○	○

Ratings ☆ ☆ ☆ ☆ ☆

Strain

Grower _____ Date _____

Acquired _____ $ _____

| Indica | Hybrid | Sativa |

☐ Flower ☐ Edible ☐ Concentrate

Symptoms Relieved

_____

_____

_____

_____

_____

Sweet

Fruity   Floral

Sour   Spicy

Earthy   Herbal

Woodsy

Notes

_____

_____

_____

_____

_____

_____

_____

Effects	Strength				
Peaceful	○	○	○	○	○
Sleepy	○	○	○	○	○
Pain Relief	○	○	○	○	○
Hungry	○	○	○	○	○
Uplifted	○	○	○	○	○
Creative	○	○	○	○	○

Ratings ☆ ☆ ☆ ☆ ☆

Strain

Grower _____ Date _____

Acquired _____ $ _____

| Indica | Hybrid | Sativa |

☐ Flower ☐ Edible ☐ Concentrate

Symptoms Relieved

_____

_____

_____

_____

_____

Sweet
Fruity   Floral
Sour   Spicy
Earthy   Herbal
Woodsy

Notes

_____

_____

_____

_____

_____

_____

_____

Effects	Strength				
Peaceful	○	○	○	○	○
Sleepy	○	○	○	○	○
Pain Relief	○	○	○	○	○
Hungry	○	○	○	○	○
Uplifted	○	○	○	○	○
Creative	○	○	○	○	○

Ratings ☆ ☆ ☆ ☆ ☆

Strain

Grower _____ Date _____

Acquired _____ $ _____

| Indica | Hybrid | Sativa |

☐ Flower ☐ Edible ☐ Concentrate

Symptoms Relieved

_____
_____
_____
_____
_____

Sweet
Fruity   Floral
Sour   Spicy
Earthy   Herbal
Woodsy

Notes

_____
_____
_____
_____
_____
_____

Effects	Strength				
Peaceful	◯	◯	◯	◯	◯
Sleepy	◯	◯	◯	◯	◯
Pain Relief	◯	◯	◯	◯	◯
Hungry	◯	◯	◯	◯	◯
Uplifted	◯	◯	◯	◯	◯
Creative	◯	◯	◯	◯	◯

Ratings ☆ ☆ ☆ ☆ ☆

Strain

Grower _____ Date _____

Acquired _____ $ _____

| Indica | Hybrid | Sativa |

☐ Flower   ☐ Edible   ☐ Concentrate

Symptoms Relieved

_____

_____

_____

_____

_____

Sweet
Fruity   Floral
Sour   Spicy
Earthy   Herbal
Woodsy

Notes

_____

_____

_____

_____

_____

_____

Effects	Strength				
Peaceful	○	○	○	○	○
Sleepy	○	○	○	○	○
Pain Relief	○	○	○	○	○
Hungry	○	○	○	○	○
Uplifted	○	○	○	○	○
Creative	○	○	○	○	○

Ratings ☆ ☆ ☆ ☆ ☆

Strain

Grower _____   Date _____

Acquired _____ $ _____

| Indica | Hybrid | Sativa |

☐ Flower   ☐ Edible   ☐ Concentrate

Symptoms Relieved

_____

_____

_____

_____

_____

Sweet
Fruity   Floral
Sour   Spicy
Earthy   Herbal
Woodsy

Notes

_____

_____

_____

_____

_____

_____

Effects	Strength				
Peaceful	○	○	○	○	○
Sleepy	○	○	○	○	○
Pain Relief	○	○	○	○	○
Hungry	○	○	○	○	○
Uplifted	○	○	○	○	○
Creative	○	○	○	○	○

Ratings ☆ ☆ ☆ ☆ ☆

Strain

Grower _____   Date _____

Acquired _____ $ _____

Indica	Hybrid	Sativa

☐ Flower   ☐ Edible   ☐ Concentrate

Symptoms Relieved

_____

_____

_____

_____

_____

Sweet

Fruity   Floral

Sour   Spicy

Earthy   Herbal

Woodsy

Notes

_____

_____

_____

_____

_____

_____

Effects	Strength				
Peaceful	○	○	○	○	○
Sleepy	○	○	○	○	○
Pain Relief	○	○	○	○	○
Hungry	○	○	○	○	○
Uplifted	○	○	○	○	○
Creative	○	○	○	○	○

Ratings ☆ ☆ ☆ ☆ ☆

Strain

Grower _____   Date _____

Acquired _____ $ _____

| Indica | Hybrid | Sativa |

☐ Flower   ☐ Edible   ☐ Concentrate

Symptoms Relieved

_____
_____
_____
_____
_____

Sweet
Fruity   Floral
Sour   Spicy
Earthy   Herbal
Woodsy

Notes

_____
_____
_____
_____
_____
_____

Effects	Strength				
Peaceful	○	○	○	○	○
Sleepy	○	○	○	○	○
Pain Relief	○	○	○	○	○
Hungry	○	○	○	○	○
Uplifted	○	○	○	○	○
Creative	○	○	○	○	○

Ratings ☆ ☆ ☆ ☆ ☆

Strain

Grower _____ Date _____

Acquired _____ $ _____

| Indica | Hybrid | Sativa |

☐ Flower   ☐ Edible   ☐ Concentrate

Symptoms Relieved

_____

_____

_____

_____

_____

Sweet
Fruity   Floral
Sour   Spicy
Earthy   Herbal
Woodsy

Notes

_____

_____

_____

_____

_____

_____

_____

Effects	Strength				
Peaceful	○	○	○	○	○
Sleepy	○	○	○	○	○
Pain Relief	○	○	○	○	○
Hungry	○	○	○	○	○
Uplifted	○	○	○	○	○
Creative	○	○	○	○	○

Ratings ☆ ☆ ☆ ☆ ☆

Strain

Grower _____ Date _____

Acquired _____ $ _____

| Indica | Hybrid | Sativa |

☐ Flower ☐ Edible ☐ Concentrate

Symptoms Relieved

_____
_____
_____
_____
_____

Sweet

Fruity   Floral

Sour   Spicy

Earthy   Herbal

Woodsy

Notes

_____
_____
_____
_____
_____
_____
_____

Effects	Strength				
Peaceful	○	○	○	○	○
Sleepy	○	○	○	○	○
Pain Relief	○	○	○	○	○
Hungry	○	○	○	○	○
Uplifted	○	○	○	○	○
Creative	○	○	○	○	○

Ratings ☆ ☆ ☆ ☆ ☆

Strain

Grower _____   Date _____

Acquired _____ $ _____

| Indica | Hybrid | Sativa |

☐ Flower   ☐ Edible   ☐ Concentrate

Symptoms Relieved

_____

_____

_____

_____

_____

Sweet
Fruity   Floral
Sour   Spicy
Earthy   Herbal
Woodsy

Notes

_____

_____

_____

_____

_____

_____

Effects	Strength
Peaceful	○ ○ ○ ○ ○
Sleepy	○ ○ ○ ○ ○
Pain Relief	○ ○ ○ ○ ○
Hungry	○ ○ ○ ○ ○
Uplifted	○ ○ ○ ○ ○
Creative	○ ○ ○ ○ ○

Ratings ☆ ☆ ☆ ☆ ☆

Strain

Grower _____ Date _____

Acquired _____ $ _____

| Indica | Hybrid | Sativa |

☐ Flower ☐ Edible ☐ Concentrate

Symptoms Relieved

_____

_____

_____

_____

_____

Sweet
Fruity   Floral
Sour   Spicy
Earthy   Herbal
Woodsy

Notes

_____

_____

_____

_____

_____

_____

Effects	Strength				
Peaceful	○	○	○	○	○
Sleepy	○	○	○	○	○
Pain Relief	○	○	○	○	○
Hungry	○	○	○	○	○
Uplifted	○	○	○	○	○
Creative	○	○	○	○	○

Ratings ☆ ☆ ☆ ☆ ☆

Strain

Grower _____   Date _____

Acquired _____ $ _____

| Indica | Hybrid | Sativa |

☐ Flower   ☐ Edible   ☐ Concentrate

Symptoms Relieved

_____

_____

_____

_____

_____

Sweet
Fruity   Floral
Sour   Spicy
Earthy   Herbal
Woodsy

Notes

_____

_____

_____

_____

_____

_____

_____

Effects	Strength
Peaceful	○ ○ ○ ○ ○
Sleepy	○ ○ ○ ○ ○
Pain Relief	○ ○ ○ ○ ○
Hungry	○ ○ ○ ○ ○
Uplifted	○ ○ ○ ○ ○
Creative	○ ○ ○ ○ ○

Ratings ☆ ☆ ☆ ☆ ☆

Strain

Grower _____ Date _____

Acquired _____ $ _____

| Indica | Hybrid | Sativa |

☐ Flower ☐ Edible ☐ Concentrate

Symptoms Relieved

_____
_____
_____
_____
_____

Sweet

Fruity   Floral

Sour   Spicy

Earthy   Herbal

Woodsy

Notes

_____
_____
_____
_____
_____
_____

Effects	Strength				
Peaceful	○	○	○	○	○
Sleepy	○	○	○	○	○
Pain Relief	○	○	○	○	○
Hungry	○	○	○	○	○
Uplifted	○	○	○	○	○
Creative	○	○	○	○	○

Ratings ☆ ☆ ☆ ☆ ☆

Strain

Grower _____ Date _____

Acquired _____ $ _____

| Indica | Hybrid | Sativa |

☐ Flower ☐ Edible ☐ Concentrate

Symptoms Relieved

_____
_____
_____
_____
_____

Sweet
Fruity   Floral
Sour   Spicy
Earthy   Herbal
Woodsy

Notes

_____
_____
_____
_____
_____
_____
_____

Effects	Strength				
Peaceful	○	○	○	○	○
Sleepy	○	○	○	○	○
Pain Relief	○	○	○	○	○
Hungry	○	○	○	○	○
Uplifted	○	○	○	○	○
Creative	○	○	○	○	○

Ratings ☆ ☆ ☆ ☆ ☆

Strain

Grower _____   Date _____

Acquired _____ $ _____

| Indica | Hybrid | Sativa |

☐ Flower   ☐ Edible   ☐ Concentrate

Symptoms Relieved

_____

_____

_____

_____

_____

Sweet
Fruity   Floral
Sour   Spicy
Earthy   Herbal
Woodsy

Notes

_____

_____

_____

_____

_____

_____

_____

Effects	Strength				
Peaceful	○	○	○	○	○
Sleepy	○	○	○	○	○
Pain Relief	○	○	○	○	○
Hungry	○	○	○	○	○
Uplifted	○	○	○	○	○
Creative	○	○	○	○	○

Ratings ☆ ☆ ☆ ☆ ☆

Strain

Grower _____   Date _____

Acquired _____ $ _____

| Indica | Hybrid | Sativa |

☐ Flower   ☐ Edible   ☐ Concentrate

Symptoms Relieved

_____

_____

_____

_____

_____

Sweet

Fruity   Floral

Sour   Spicy

Earthy   Herbal

Woodsy

Notes

_____

_____

_____

_____

_____

_____

_____

Effects	Strength				
Peaceful	○	○	○	○	○
Sleepy	○	○	○	○	○
Pain Relief	○	○	○	○	○
Hungry	○	○	○	○	○
Uplifted	○	○	○	○	○
Creative	○	○	○	○	○

Ratings ☆ ☆ ☆ ☆ ☆

Strain

Grower _____ Date _____

Acquired _____ $ _____

| Indica | Hybrid | Sativa |

☐ Flower   ☐ Edible   ☐ Concentrate

Symptoms Relieved

_____
_____
_____
_____
_____

Sweet
Fruity   Floral
Sour   Spicy
Earthy   Herbal
Woodsy

Notes

_____
_____
_____
_____
_____
_____

Effects	Strength				
Peaceful	○	○	○	○	○
Sleepy	○	○	○	○	○
Pain Relief	○	○	○	○	○
Hungry	○	○	○	○	○
Uplifted	○	○	○	○	○
Creative	○	○	○	○	○

Ratings ☆ ☆ ☆ ☆ ☆

Strain

Grower _____ Date _____

Acquired _____ $ _____

| Indica | Hybrid | Sativa |

☐ Flower   ☐ Edible   ☐ Concentrate

Symptoms Relieved

_____

_____

_____

_____

_____

Sweet
Fruity   Floral
Sour   Spicy
Earthy   Herbal
Woodsy

Notes

_____

_____

_____

_____

_____

_____

_____

Effects	Strength				
Peaceful	○	○	○	○	○
Sleepy	○	○	○	○	○
Pain Relief	○	○	○	○	○
Hungry	○	○	○	○	○
Uplifted	○	○	○	○	○
Creative	○	○	○	○	○

Ratings ☆ ☆ ☆ ☆ ☆

Strain

Grower _____ Date _____

Acquired _____ $ _____

Indica	Hybrid	Sativa

☐ Flower ☐ Edible ☐ Concentrate

Symptoms Relieved

_____

_____

_____

_____

_____

Sweet
Fruity   Floral
Sour   Spicy
Earthy   Herbal
Woodsy

Notes

_____

_____

_____

_____

_____

_____

Effects	Strength				
Peaceful	○	○	○	○	○
Sleepy	○	○	○	○	○
Pain Relief	○	○	○	○	○
Hungry	○	○	○	○	○
Uplifted	○	○	○	○	○
Creative	○	○	○	○	○

Ratings ☆ ☆ ☆ ☆ ☆

Strain

Grower _____   Date _____

Acquired _____ $ _____

| Indica | Hybrid | Sativa |

☐ Flower   ☐ Edible   ☐ Concentrate

Symptoms Relieved

_____

_____

_____

_____

_____

Sweet
Fruity   Floral
Sour   Spicy
Earthy   Herbal
Woodsy

Notes

_____

_____

_____

_____

_____

_____

_____

Effects	Strength				
Peaceful	○	○	○	○	○
Sleepy	○	○	○	○	○
Pain Relief	○	○	○	○	○
Hungry	○	○	○	○	○
Uplifted	○	○	○	○	○
Creative	○	○	○	○	○

Ratings ☆ ☆ ☆ ☆ ☆

Strain

Grower _____ Date _____

Acquired _____ $ _____

| Indica | Hybrid | Sativa |

☐ Flower ☐ Edible ☐ Concentrate

Symptoms Relieved

_____
_____
_____
_____
_____

Sweet
Fruity   Floral
Sour   Spicy
Earthy   Herbal
Woodsy

Notes

_____
_____
_____
_____
_____
_____
_____

Effects	Strength				
Peaceful	○	○	○	○	○
Sleepy	○	○	○	○	○
Pain Relief	○	○	○	○	○
Hungry	○	○	○	○	○
Uplifted	○	○	○	○	○
Creative	○	○	○	○	○

Ratings ☆ ☆ ☆ ☆ ☆

Strain

Grower _____   Date _____

Acquired _____ $ _____

| Indica | Hybrid | Sativa |

☐ Flower ☐ Edible ☐ Concentrate

Symptoms Relieved

_____
_____
_____
_____
_____

Sweet
Fruity   Floral
Sour   Spicy
Earthy   Herbal
Woodsy

Notes

_____
_____
_____
_____
_____
_____
_____

Effects	Strength				
Peaceful	○	○	○	○	○
Sleepy	○	○	○	○	○
Pain Relief	○	○	○	○	○
Hungry	○	○	○	○	○
Uplifted	○	○	○	○	○
Creative	○	○	○	○	○

Ratings ☆ ☆ ☆ ☆ ☆

Strain

Grower _____ Date _____

Acquired _____ $ _____

| Indica | Hybrid | Sativa |

☐ Flower   ☐ Edible   ☐ Concentrate

Symptoms Relieved

_____

_____

_____

_____

_____

Sweet
Fruity   Floral
Sour   Spicy
Earthy   Herbal
Woodsy

Notes

_____

_____

_____

_____

_____

_____

Effects	Strength				
Peaceful	○	○	○	○	○
Sleepy	○	○	○	○	○
Pain Relief	○	○	○	○	○
Hungry	○	○	○	○	○
Uplifted	○	○	○	○	○
Creative	○	○	○	○	○

Ratings ☆ ☆ ☆ ☆ ☆

Strain

Grower _____ Date _____

Acquired _____ $ _____

| Indica | Hybrid | Sativa |

☐ Flower ☐ Edible ☐ Concentrate

Symptoms Relieved

_____

_____

_____

_____

_____

Sweet

Fruity   Floral

Sour   Spicy

Earthy   Herbal

Woodsy

Notes

_____

_____

_____

_____

_____

_____

_____

Effects	Strength				
Peaceful	○	○	○	○	○
Sleepy	○	○	○	○	○
Pain Relief	○	○	○	○	○
Hungry	○	○	○	○	○
Uplifted	○	○	○	○	○
Creative	○	○	○	○	○

Ratings ☆ ☆ ☆ ☆ ☆

Strain

Grower _____   Date _____

Acquired _____ $ _____

Indica	Hybrid	Sativa

☐ Flower   ☐ Edible   ☐ Concentrate

Symptoms Relieved

_____

_____

_____

_____

_____

Sweet
Fruity   Floral
Sour   Spicy
Earthy   Herbal
Woodsy

Notes

_____

_____

_____

_____

_____

_____

_____

Effects	Strength				
Peaceful	○	○	○	○	○
Sleepy	○	○	○	○	○
Pain Relief	○	○	○	○	○
Hungry	○	○	○	○	○
Uplifted	○	○	○	○	○
Creative	○	○	○	○	○

Ratings ☆ ☆ ☆ ☆ ☆

Strain

Grower _____   Date _____

Acquired _____ $ _____

Indica	Hybrid	Sativa

☐ Flower   ☐ Edible   ☐ Concentrate

Symptoms Relieved

_____

_____

_____

_____

_____

Sweet
Fruity   Floral
Sour   Spicy
Earthy   Herbal
Woodsy

Notes

_____

_____

_____

_____

_____

_____

Effects	Strength				
Peaceful	○	○	○	○	○
Sleepy	○	○	○	○	○
Pain Relief	○	○	○	○	○
Hungry	○	○	○	○	○
Uplifted	○	○	○	○	○
Creative	○	○	○	○	○

Ratings ☆ ☆ ☆ ☆ ☆

Strain

Grower _____ Date _____

Acquired _____ $ _____

| Indica | Hybrid | Sativa |

☐ Flower ☐ Edible ☐ Concentrate

Symptoms Relieved

_____
_____
_____
_____
_____

Sweet
Fruity   Floral
Sour   Spicy
Earthy   Herbal
Woodsy

Notes

_____
_____
_____
_____
_____
_____
_____

Effects	Strength				
Peaceful	○	○	○	○	○
Sleepy	○	○	○	○	○
Pain Relief	○	○	○	○	○
Hungry	○	○	○	○	○
Uplifted	○	○	○	○	○
Creative	○	○	○	○	○

Ratings ☆ ☆ ☆ ☆ ☆

Strain

Grower _____ Date _____

Acquired _____ $ _____

Indica	Hybrid	Sativa

☐ Flower   ☐ Edible   ☐ Concentrate

Symptoms Relieved

_____

_____

_____

_____

_____

Sweet

Fruity   Floral

Sour   Spicy

Earthy   Herbal

Woodsy

Notes

_____

_____

_____

_____

_____

_____

_____

Effects	Strength				
Peaceful	○	○	○	○	○
Sleepy	○	○	○	○	○
Pain Relief	○	○	○	○	○
Hungry	○	○	○	○	○
Uplifted	○	○	○	○	○
Creative	○	○	○	○	○

Ratings ☆ ☆ ☆ ☆ ☆

Strain

Grower _____   Date _____

Acquired _____ $ _____

| Indica | Hybrid | Sativa |

☐ Flower   ☐ Edible   ☐ Concentrate

Symptoms Relieved

_____

_____

_____

_____

_____

Sweet
Fruity   Floral
Sour   Spicy
Earthy   Herbal
Woodsy

Notes

_____

_____

_____

_____

_____

_____

Effects	Strength				
Peaceful	○	○	○	○	○
Sleepy	○	○	○	○	○
Pain Relief	○	○	○	○	○
Hungry	○	○	○	○	○
Uplifted	○	○	○	○	○
Creative	○	○	○	○	○

Ratings ☆ ☆ ☆ ☆ ☆

Strain

Grower _____   Date _____

Acquired _____ $ _____

| Indica | Hybrid | Sativa |

☐ Flower   ☐ Edible   ☐ Concentrate

Symptoms Relieved

_____

_____

_____

_____

_____

Sweet
Fruity   Floral
Sour   Spicy
Earthy   Herbal
Woodsy

Notes

_____

_____

_____

_____

_____

_____

Effects	Strength				
Peaceful	○	○	○	○	○
Sleepy	○	○	○	○	○
Pain Relief	○	○	○	○	○
Hungry	○	○	○	○	○
Uplifted	○	○	○	○	○
Creative	○	○	○	○	○

Ratings ☆ ☆ ☆ ☆ ☆

Strain

Grower _____ Date _____

Acquired _____ $ _____

| Indica | Hybrid | Sativa |

☐ Flower   ☐ Edible   ☐ Concentrate

Symptoms Relieved

_____
_____
_____
_____
_____

Sweet
Fruity   Floral
Sour   Spicy
Earthy   Herbal
Woodsy

Notes

_____
_____
_____
_____
_____
_____
_____

Effects	Strength				
Peaceful	○	○	○	○	○
Sleepy	○	○	○	○	○
Pain Relief	○	○	○	○	○
Hungry	○	○	○	○	○
Uplifted	○	○	○	○	○
Creative	○	○	○	○	○

Ratings ☆ ☆ ☆ ☆ ☆

Strain

Grower _____ Date _____

Acquired _____ $ _____

| Indica | Hybrid | Sativa |

☐ Flower ☐ Edible ☐ Concentrate

Symptoms Relieved

_____

_____

_____

_____

_____

Sweet

Fruity   Floral

Sour   Spicy

Earthy   Herbal

Woodsy

Notes

_____

_____

_____

_____

_____

_____

_____

Effects	Strength				
Peaceful	○	○	○	○	○
Sleepy	○	○	○	○	○
Pain Relief	○	○	○	○	○
Hungry	○	○	○	○	○
Uplifted	○	○	○	○	○
Creative	○	○	○	○	○

Ratings ☆ ☆ ☆ ☆ ☆

Strain

Grower _____   Date _____

Acquired _____ $ _____

| Indica | Hybrid | Sativa |

☐ Flower   ☐ Edible   ☐ Concentrate

Symptoms Relieved

_____
_____
_____
_____
_____

Sweet
Fruity   Floral
Sour   Spicy
Earthy   Herbal
Woodsy

Notes

_____
_____
_____
_____
_____
_____
_____

Effects	Strength				
Peaceful	○	○	○	○	○
Sleepy	○	○	○	○	○
Pain Relief	○	○	○	○	○
Hungry	○	○	○	○	○
Uplifted	○	○	○	○	○
Creative	○	○	○	○	○

Ratings ☆ ☆ ☆ ☆ ☆

Strain

Grower _____ Date _____

Acquired _____ $ _____

Indica	Hybrid	Sativa

☐ Flower ☐ Edible ☐ Concentrate

Symptoms Relieved

_____

_____

_____

_____

_____

Sweet
Fruity   Floral
Sour   Spicy
Earthy   Herbal
Woodsy

Notes

_____

_____

_____

_____

_____

_____

Effects	Strength				
Peaceful	○	○	○	○	○
Sleepy	○	○	○	○	○
Pain Relief	○	○	○	○	○
Hungry	○	○	○	○	○
Uplifted	○	○	○	○	○
Creative	○	○	○	○	○

Ratings ☆ ☆ ☆ ☆ ☆

Strain

Grower _____   Date _____

Acquired _____ $ _____

| Indica | Hybrid | Sativa |

☐ Flower   ☐ Edible   ☐ Concentrate

Symptoms Relieved

_____

_____

_____

_____

_____

Sweet

Fruity   **Floral**

Sour   **Spicy**

Earthy   **Herbal**

Woodsy

Notes

_____

_____

_____

_____

_____

_____

Effects	Strength				
Peaceful	○	○	○	○	○
Sleepy	○	○	○	○	○
Pain Relief	○	○	○	○	○
Hungry	○	○	○	○	○
Uplifted	○	○	○	○	○
Creative	○	○	○	○	○

Ratings ☆ ☆ ☆ ☆ ☆

Strain

Grower _____   Date _____

Acquired _____ $ _____

| Indica | Hybrid | Sativa |

☐ Flower   ☐ Edible   ☐ Concentrate

Symptoms Relieved

_____

_____

_____

_____

_____

Sweet
Fruity   Floral
Sour   Spicy
Earthy   Herbal
Woodsy

Notes

_____

_____

_____

_____

_____

_____

Effects	Strength				
Peaceful	○	○	○	○	○
Sleepy	○	○	○	○	○
Pain Relief	○	○	○	○	○
Hungry	○	○	○	○	○
Uplifted	○	○	○	○	○
Creative	○	○	○	○	○

Ratings ☆ ☆ ☆ ☆ ☆

Strain

Grower _____ Date _____

Acquired _____ $ _____

| Indica | Hybrid | Sativa |

☐ Flower ☐ Edible ☐ Concentrate

Symptoms Relieved

_____
_____
_____
_____
_____

Sweet
Fruity   Floral
Sour   Spicy
Earthy   Herbal
Woodsy

Notes

_____
_____
_____
_____
_____
_____

Effects	Strength				
Peaceful	○	○	○	○	○
Sleepy	○	○	○	○	○
Pain Relief	○	○	○	○	○
Hungry	○	○	○	○	○
Uplifted	○	○	○	○	○
Creative	○	○	○	○	○

Ratings ☆ ☆ ☆ ☆ ☆

Strain

Grower _____   Date _____

Acquired _____ $ _____

| Indica | Hybrid | Sativa |

☐ Flower   ☐ Edible   ☐ Concentrate

Symptoms Relieved

_____

_____

_____

_____

_____

Sweet
Fruity
Floral
Sour
Spicy
Earthy
Herbal
Woodsy

Notes

_____

_____

_____

_____

_____

_____

_____

Effects	Strength				
Peaceful	○	○	○	○	○
Sleepy	○	○	○	○	○
Pain Relief	○	○	○	○	○
Hungry	○	○	○	○	○
Uplifted	○	○	○	○	○
Creative	○	○	○	○	○

Ratings ☆ ☆ ☆ ☆ ☆

Strain

Grower _____ Date _____

Acquired _____ $ _____

Indica	Hybrid	Sativa

☐ Flower ☐ Edible ☐ Concentrate

Symptoms Relieved

_____

_____

_____

_____

_____

Sweet
Fruity   Floral
Sour   Spicy
Earthy   Herbal
Woodsy

Notes

_____

_____

_____

_____

_____

_____

Effects	Strength				
Peaceful	○	○	○	○	○
Sleepy	○	○	○	○	○
Pain Relief	○	○	○	○	○
Hungry	○	○	○	○	○
Uplifted	○	○	○	○	○
Creative	○	○	○	○	○

Ratings ☆ ☆ ☆ ☆ ☆

Strain

Grower _____   Date _____

Acquired _____ $ _____

Indica	Hybrid	Sativa

☐ Flower ☐ Edible ☐ Concentrate

Symptoms Relieved

_____

_____

_____

_____

_____

Sweet
Fruity   Floral
Sour   Spicy
Earthy   Herbal
Woodsy

Notes

_____

_____

_____

_____

_____

_____

_____

Effects	Strength				
Peaceful	○	○	○	○	○
Sleepy	○	○	○	○	○
Pain Relief	○	○	○	○	○
Hungry	○	○	○	○	○
Uplifted	○	○	○	○	○
Creative	○	○	○	○	○

Ratings ☆ ☆ ☆ ☆ ☆

Strain

Grower _____   Date _____

Acquired _____ $ _____

Indica	Hybrid	Sativa

☐ Flower   ☐ Edible   ☐ Concentrate

Symptoms Relieved

_____

_____

_____

_____

_____

Sweet
Fruity   Floral
Sour   Spicy
Earthy   Herbal
Woodsy

Notes

_____

_____

_____

_____

_____

_____

_____

Effects	Strength				
Peaceful	○	○	○	○	○
Sleepy	○	○	○	○	○
Pain Relief	○	○	○	○	○
Hungry	○	○	○	○	○
Uplifted	○	○	○	○	○
Creative	○	○	○	○	○

Ratings ☆ ☆ ☆ ☆ ☆

Strain

Grower _____ Date _____

Acquired _____ $ _____

| Indica | Hybrid | Sativa |

☐ Flower ☐ Edible ☐ Concentrate

Symptoms Relieved

_____

_____

_____

_____

_____

Sweet
Fruity   Floral
Sour   Spicy
Earthy   Herbal
Woodsy

Notes

_____

_____

_____

_____

_____

_____

Effects	**Strength**				
Peaceful	○	○	○	○	○
Sleepy	○	○	○	○	○
Pain Relief	○	○	○	○	○
Hungry	○	○	○	○	○
Uplifted	○	○	○	○	○
Creative	○	○	○	○	○

Ratings ☆ ☆ ☆ ☆ ☆

Strain

Grower _____ Date _____

Acquired _____ $ _____

| Indica | Hybrid | Sativa |

☐ Flower ☐ Edible ☐ Concentrate

Symptoms Relieved

_____

_____

_____

_____

_____

Sweet

Fruity   Floral

Sour   Spicy

Earthy   Herbal

Woodsy

Notes

_____

_____

_____

_____

_____

_____

_____

Effects	Strength				
Peaceful	○	○	○	○	○
Sleepy	○	○	○	○	○
Pain Relief	○	○	○	○	○
Hungry	○	○	○	○	○
Uplifted	○	○	○	○	○
Creative	○	○	○	○	○

Ratings ☆ ☆ ☆ ☆ ☆

Strain

Grower _____ Date _____

Acquired _____ $ _____

| Indica | Hybrid | Sativa |

☐ Flower   ☐ Edible   ☐ Concentrate

Symptoms Relieved

_____

_____

_____

_____

_____

Sweet
Fruity   Floral
Sour   Spicy
Earthy   Herbal
Woodsy

Notes

_____

_____

_____

_____

_____

_____

Effects	Strength
Peaceful	○ ○ ○ ○ ○
Sleepy	○ ○ ○ ○ ○
Pain Relief	○ ○ ○ ○ ○
Hungry	○ ○ ○ ○ ○
Uplifted	○ ○ ○ ○ ○
Creative	○ ○ ○ ○ ○

Ratings ☆ ☆ ☆ ☆ ☆

Strain

Grower _____   Date _____

Acquired _____ $ _____

| Indica | Hybrid | Sativa |

☐ Flower ☐ Edible ☐ Concentrate

Symptoms Relieved

_____

_____

_____

_____

_____

Sweet

Fruity   Floral

Sour   Spicy

Earthy   Herbal

Woodsy

Notes

_____

_____

_____

_____

_____

_____

_____

Effects	Strength
Peaceful	○ ○ ○ ○ ○
Sleepy	○ ○ ○ ○ ○
Pain Relief	○ ○ ○ ○ ○
Hungry	○ ○ ○ ○ ○
Uplifted	○ ○ ○ ○ ○
Creative	○ ○ ○ ○ ○

Ratings ☆ ☆ ☆ ☆ ☆

Strain

Grower _____ Date _____

Acquired _____ $ _____

| Indica | Hybrid | Sativa |

☐ Flower ☐ Edible ☐ Concentrate

Symptoms Relieved

_____

_____

_____

_____

_____

Sweet

Fruity   Floral

Sour   Spicy

Earthy   Herbal

Woodsy

Notes

_____

_____

_____

_____

_____

_____

Effects	Strength				
Peaceful	○	○	○	○	○
Sleepy	○	○	○	○	○
Pain Relief	○	○	○	○	○
Hungry	○	○	○	○	○
Uplifted	○	○	○	○	○
Creative	○	○	○	○	○

Ratings ☆ ☆ ☆ ☆ ☆

Strain

Grower _____   Date _____

Acquired _____ $ _____

| Indica | Hybrid | Sativa |

☐ Flower   ☐ Edible   ☐ Concentrate

Symptoms Relieved

_____

_____

_____

_____

_____

Sweet

Fruity   Floral

Sour   Spicy

Earthy   Herbal

Woodsy

Notes

_____

_____

_____

_____

_____

_____

Effects	**Strength**				
Peaceful	○	○	○	○	○
Sleepy	○	○	○	○	○
Pain Relief	○	○	○	○	○
Hungry	○	○	○	○	○
Uplifted	○	○	○	○	○
Creative	○	○	○	○	○

Ratings ☆ ☆ ☆ ☆ ☆

Strain

Grower _____ Date _____

Acquired _____ $ _____

| Indica | Hybrid | Sativa |

☐ Flower ☐ Edible ☐ Concentrate

Symptoms Relieved

_____

_____

_____

_____

_____

Sweet
Fruity   Floral
Sour   Spicy
Earthy   Herbal
Woodsy

Notes

_____

_____

_____

_____

_____

_____

Effects	Strength				
Peaceful	○	○	○	○	○
Sleepy	○	○	○	○	○
Pain Relief	○	○	○	○	○
Hungry	○	○	○	○	○
Uplifted	○	○	○	○	○
Creative	○	○	○	○	○

Ratings ☆ ☆ ☆ ☆ ☆

Strain

Grower _____   Date _____

Acquired _____ $ _____

| Indica | Hybrid | Sativa |

☐ Flower   ☐ Edible   ☐ Concentrate

Symptoms Relieved

_____

_____

_____

_____

_____

Sweet
Fruity
Floral
Sour
Spicy
Earthy
Herbal
Woodsy

Notes

_____

_____

_____

_____

_____

_____

Effects	Strength				
Peaceful	○	○	○	○	○
Sleepy	○	○	○	○	○
Pain Relief	○	○	○	○	○
Hungry	○	○	○	○	○
Uplifted	○	○	○	○	○
Creative	○	○	○	○	○

Ratings ☆ ☆ ☆ ☆ ☆

Strain

Grower _____   Date _____

Acquired _____ $ _____

| Indica | Hybrid | Sativa |

☐ Flower   ☐ Edible   ☐ Concentrate

Symptoms Relieved

_____

_____

_____

_____

_____

Sweet

Fruity   Floral

Sour   Spicy

Earthy   Herbal

Woodsy

Notes

_____

_____

_____

_____

_____

_____

Effects	Strength				
Peaceful	◯	◯	◯	◯	◯
Sleepy	◯	◯	◯	◯	◯
Pain Relief	◯	◯	◯	◯	◯
Hungry	◯	◯	◯	◯	◯
Uplifted	◯	◯	◯	◯	◯
Creative	◯	◯	◯	◯	◯

Ratings ☆ ☆ ☆ ☆ ☆

Strain

Grower _____   Date _____

Acquired _____ $ _____

Indica	Hybrid	Sativa

☐ Flower   ☐ Edible   ☐ Concentrate

Symptoms Relieved

_____

_____

_____

_____

_____

Sweet
Fruity   Floral
Sour   Spicy
Earthy   Herbal
Woodsy

Notes

_____

_____

_____

_____

_____

_____

_____

Effects	Strength				
Peaceful	○	○	○	○	○
Sleepy	○	○	○	○	○
Pain Relief	○	○	○	○	○
Hungry	○	○	○	○	○
Uplifted	○	○	○	○	○
Creative	○	○	○	○	○

Ratings ☆ ☆ ☆ ☆ ☆

Strain

Grower _____ Date _____

Acquired _____ $ _____

| Indica | Hybrid | Sativa |

☐ Flower ☐ Edible ☐ Concentrate

Symptoms Relieved

_____

_____

_____

_____

_____

Sweet

Fruity   Floral

Sour   Spicy

Earthy   Herbal

Woodsy

Notes

_____

_____

_____

_____

_____

_____

_____

Effects	Strength
Peaceful	○ ○ ○ ○ ○
Sleepy	○ ○ ○ ○ ○
Pain Relief	○ ○ ○ ○ ○
Hungry	○ ○ ○ ○ ○
Uplifted	○ ○ ○ ○ ○
Creative	○ ○ ○ ○ ○

Ratings ☆ ☆ ☆ ☆ ☆

Strain

Grower _____ Date _____

Acquired _____ $ _____

Indica	Hybrid	Sativa

☐ Flower ☐ Edible ☐ Concentrate

Symptoms Relieved

_____

_____

_____

_____

_____

Sweet

Fruity   Floral

Sour   Spicy

Earthy   Herbal

Woodsy

Notes

_____

_____

_____

_____

_____

_____

_____

Effects	Strength				
Peaceful	○	○	○	○	○
Sleepy	○	○	○	○	○
Pain Relief	○	○	○	○	○
Hungry	○	○	○	○	○
Uplifted	○	○	○	○	○
Creative	○	○	○	○	○

Ratings ☆ ☆ ☆ ☆ ☆

Strain

Grower _____   Date _____

Acquired _____ $ _____

Indica	Hybrid	Sativa

☐ Flower ☐ Edible ☐ Concentrate

Symptoms Relieved

_____

_____

_____

_____

_____

Sweet

Fruity   Floral

Sour   Spicy

Earthy   Herbal

Woodsy

Notes

_____

_____

_____

_____

_____

_____

Effects	Strength				
Peaceful	○	○	○	○	○
Sleepy	○	○	○	○	○
Pain Relief	○	○	○	○	○
Hungry	○	○	○	○	○
Uplifted	○	○	○	○	○
Creative	○	○	○	○	○

Ratings ☆ ☆ ☆ ☆ ☆

Strain

Grower _____ Date _____

Acquired _____ $ _____

Indica	Hybrid	Sativa

☐ Flower   ☐ Edible   ☐ Concentrate

Symptoms Relieved

_____

_____

_____

_____

_____

Sweet

Fruity   Floral

Sour   Spicy

Earthy   Herbal

Woodsy

Notes

_____

_____

_____

_____

_____

_____

Effects	Strength				
Peaceful	○	○	○	○	○
Sleepy	○	○	○	○	○
Pain Relief	○	○	○	○	○
Hungry	○	○	○	○	○
Uplifted	○	○	○	○	○
Creative	○	○	○	○	○

Ratings ☆ ☆ ☆ ☆ ☆

Strain

Grower _____   Date _____

Acquired _____ $ _____

| Indica | Hybrid | Sativa |

☐ Flower   ☐ Edible   ☐ Concentrate

Symptoms Relieved

_____

_____

_____

_____

_____

Sweet
Fruity   Floral
Sour   Spicy
Earthy   Herbal
Woodsy

Notes

_____

_____

_____

_____

_____

_____

_____

Effects	Strength				
Peaceful	○	○	○	○	○
Sleepy	○	○	○	○	○
Pain Relief	○	○	○	○	○
Hungry	○	○	○	○	○
Uplifted	○	○	○	○	○
Creative	○	○	○	○	○

Ratings ☆ ☆ ☆ ☆ ☆

Made in the USA
Monee, IL
07 July 2026

56550176R00059